Weight Loss Surgery

The Ultimate Introductory Guide to Bariatric Surgery, Including Gastric Bypass, Sleeve And Diet

presentation of the information is without contract or any type of guarantee assurance.

The trademarks that are used are without any consent, and the publication of the trademark is without permission or backing by the trademark owner. All trademarks and brands within this book are for clarifying purposes only and are the owned by the owners themselves, not affiliated with this document.

Table Of Contents

Introduction

First off, I really want to thank you for downloading this book. The pages in this book were developed through years of experiences that I have gone through, as well as what has proven to work for others that I have talked to and researched. I also want to congratulate you for taking the time to understand weight loss surgery and possibly leading a healthier lifestyle.

This short e-book discusses the advantages and side effects of different forms of weight loss surgery. Hopefully after understanding these options, you will have a better idea of whether or not you want to undergo surgery. The benefits outlined here are taken from years of collective experiences and testimonials backed by scientific research.

I can guarantee that you will find this book useful if you make sure to implement what you learn in the following pages. The important thing is that you IMPLEMENT what you learn. A change in diet and lifestyle is not conquered overnight but the important thing to remember, is that it is definitely possible for you to make the change over time. What I am giving you is the information you need to get started and the guidelines you will need to make that journey.

I recommend that you take notes while you are reading the book. This will ensure that you get the most out of the information in here. I want you to feel that you made a purchase that is worth your money and I want you to look over the notes of this book even after you've finished reading it. The notes will help you to pinpoint exactly what you need to implement and by writing things down, you will be able to recall specifics and how to handle certain situations when they arise.

Lastly, remember that everything in this book has been compiled through research, my own experiences, as well as the experiences of others, so feel free to question what you have read in this book. I encourage you to do your own research on the things that you want to look deeper into. There are many myths created by supplement and pharmaceutical companies, mainly because there is profit to be made off of ignorant consumers. You must be aware of what is true and false and that is one of the reasons why I created this book.

The more you understand your own health and body, the better off you'll be. Weight loss surgery will take some preparation and planning on your part, but you can do it! So remember to read with confidence and an open mind!

Chapter 1:

Facts About Obesity and Weight Loss

When it comes to weight, how much is too much, exactly? The best way to measure this (as of now) is by using something called the body mass index, or BMI. If a person's BMI is measured to be between 25 and 29.9 then that person is classified as overweight. But if their BMI reaches 30 or more, then that person is classified as obese.

Weighing too much can put you at risk of certain health conditions and diseases, such as high blood pressure, stroke, heart disease, type 2 diabetes, gallbladder disease, osteoarthritis, colon cancer, breast cancer, and depression, among many others. On the other hand, increased physical activity and switching to a healthier and controlled diet can greatly improve anyone's health conditions.

What if diet and exercise do not work? What other options do you have?

A more natural way of losing weight is undoubtedly preferred and is more advisable. But there are also certain things that you can take to help you fight obesity. This includes FDA approved medicines like Sibutramine and Orlistat. Orlistat works by preventing the body from absorbing fat from food. On the other hand, Sibutamine works by suppressing a person's appetite.

These FDA approved medicines are recommended for those whose BMI is 30 or higher. They are also recommended for people with a BMI of 27 or higher, who are experiencing health problems related to carrying excess weight. A word of caution however, these medicines do not work magically by themselves.

If you want results, you are supposed to take them with a healthy diet and an appropriate exercise program. Self medicating is strongly discouraged. Regardless, make sure to talk to your doctor first so that you know the benefits and side effects.

Among the few things you should know, Orlistat can possibly cause oily stool leakage, gas, cramps, and diarrhea. A good way to prevent such side effects is to stick to a low fat diet. Since consuming Orlistat also carries the possibility of inhibiting vitamin absorption, taking a multi-vitamin supplement may also be a good idea.

Sibutramine on the other hand, may cause an increased heart rate and blood pressure. This means that people with heart problems and high blood pressure should avoid taking this weight loss medicine.

The Surgical Option

It is also not uncommon for people with weight loss problems to go through drastic measures to get into shape. An even faster way to lose the extra pounds is through surgery.

Weight loss surgery, or bariatric surgery, is a common procedure performed to assist people in their weight loss journey. Unlike liposuction, which focuses on specific problem areas in the body and only caters to individuals who are close to their ideal weight, bariatric surgery is specifically for those who are in an unhealthy weight range.

For some patients, the stomach size may be reduced by using a gastric band. In other cases, a portion of the stomach may be removed altogether. Still, in others, the small intestine is re-routed to a smaller stomach pouch. The way the procedure will be done depends on your own consultation with your doctor.

According to studies, weight loss surgery can help significantly with long term weight loss. It is also proven to be helpful for patients recovering from diabetes. Through bariatric surgery, a person's risk for cardiovascular problems may also be reduced. Although surgery may seem like an extreme measure to treat obesity, it does prove to be effective in many people, especially in reducing mortality rates by 17 percent among obese people.

Chapter 2:

Is Bariatric Surgery for You?

The first form of weight loss surgery was introduced in the 1950s, however, at that time it was a relatively uncommon treatment and not taken very seriously by the general public. But in recent years, the idea of weight loss surgery has gained momentum and has reached a surprising level of popularity.

For instance, in the United States, the number of patients who have undergone bariatric surgery has grown from 13,000 in 1998 to around 121,000 in 2003. And according to the American Society for Metabolic and Bariatric Surgery, the number of patients further increased to 220,000 in 2008.

However, considering the number of obese people in the United States, these figures are still nowhere near the maximum. In the United States, only 1 percent of the obese population has had the treatment done, despite the promising results of this procedure.

How Does It Work?

Despite many doubters, bariatric surgery can indeed result in dramatic weight loss and there is medical research that backs up the effectiveness of this procedure. There are two basic ways by which bariatric surgery can work.

First off, the surgery works to limit a person's food intake by reducing the amount of food the stomach can hold. Secondly, it can prevent the digestive system from absorbing fats and nutrients from food.

Before you decide if weight loss surgery is right for you, it is important that you understand the benefits and risks that are involved in this procedure.

On the Upside:

Pros of Bariatric Surgery

There are two main benefits to having weight loss surgery. First off, weight loss is almost guaranteed. In fact, most individuals who undergo this kind of procedure experience weight loss immediately after the surgery.

This continuous weight loss usually occurs pretty steadily for up to two years after the surgery. In some cases, patients regain the weight, if they become undisciplined in their lifestyle. However, with proper care and discipline, it is possible to keep off the lost weight for good.

Another major advantage to bariatric surgery is that it can greatly improve obesity related conditions such as diabetes. According to research, the surgery proves to be more effective in controlling a patient's blood sugar level than some forms of medication can. And this does not only depend on the amount of weight lost after the procedure, which is definitely good news for people who happen to be obese and diabetic.

On the Downside:

Cons of Bariatric Surgery

Bariatric surgery should not be viewed as a magical solution. Since we are talking about a medical procedure here, you should also expect a certain amount of risk. There are also some side effects that you should be aware of.

For one, there is the risk of complications. There are patients who have experienced complications from the surgery, which include infections and abdominal hernias. The staple line that is used to reduce the size of the stomach may also break down in some cases.

Also, when the stomach starts to return to its normal size, there is a possibility of experiencing stretched stomach outlets. These are only some of the possible complications that may occur after the surgery, and they would require follow up treatments for correction.

Your chosen surgeon should be able to help prevent the occurrence of such complications as long as you follow the provided instructions before and after the surgery.

Another possible risk is the development of nutritional deficiencies, including anemia, metabolic bone disease, and osteoporosis. Some procedures work to prevent the absorption of nutrients from food; while this may lead to weight loss, it can also lead to nutritional deficiencies. This is why a surgeon will usually recommend vitamin and mineral supplements to make up for what your body may not be able to get from the foods you eat.

For malabsorptive surgery specifically, patients may experience what is referred to as the "dumping syndrome." This can involve weakness, faintness, sweating, and nausea, among others. Dumping syndrome occurs when the elements from the stomach move too quickly through the small intestine. Patients with dumping syndrome may also experience diarrhea after meals.

On the other hand, restrictive types of surgery may cause vomiting. When a patient eats and the food is not chewed well, the small stomach may become overly stretched. As a result, the stomach will force the food out.

Individuals who undergo gastric surgery also face the risk of developing gallstones. This is a common condition among people who lose a substantial amount of weight. However, such can be prevented with the help of supplemental bile salts. This is usually prescribed 6 months after the procedure.

Women who are considering weight loss surgery must avoid getting pregnant until their weight is stable. This is because nutritional deficiencies and the dramatic weight loss can be dangerous to a developing fetus.

Other common side effects of bariatric surgery include vomiting, nausea, diarrhea, bloating, increased gas, excessive sweating, and dizziness. But most risks and side effects of surgery can be prevented, provided that patients apply the necessary lifestyle changes and comply with the right diet, proper vitamin and mineral supplementation, and exercise, along with regular visits to the doctor for close monitoring.

Are You a Viable Candidate for Bariatric Surgery?

This surgery may be increasingly popular, however, weight loss surgery is still considered a drastic measure of losing weight. Before you even consider surgery, you need an honest personal evaluation of your situation before visiting your doctor. Ask yourself the following questions:

Have I honestly exerted time and effort so that I could lose weight?

Have I truly given dieting and exercise a shot?

Were my efforts enough?

Have I completed at least a year of following a medically supervised program for weight loss?

In case I go through the procedure, will my insurance be able to cover the expenses?

Am I prepared physically, emotionally and psychologically for this?

Do I have a support system to help me out during my recovery from surgery?

It is important to understand that this kind of operation is not for everyone. Weight loss surgery is only recommended for certain individuals who meet the following criteria:

One, to be a viable candidate for bariatric surgery, you must have a BMI of 40 or more. This means that you must be at least a hundred pounds heavier than your ideal weight if you are male, and 80 pounds overweight if you are a female.

If your BMI is below 40 but not less than 35, you must be dealing with a serious weight related health problem in order to qualify. This may include type 2 diabetes, heart disease, severe sleep apnea, and/or high cholesterol.

Two, doctors only recommend this procedure for individuals who have made serious attempts to lose weight through non surgical methods. This means you must have tried dieting and exercise programs before you will even be considered a viable candidate for this procedure.

Finally, it is crucial that you have a complete understanding of the risks involved in this kind of procedure. You must have a strong motivation so that you can fully prepare yourself physically, emotionally and psychologically.

Consider bariatric surgery as a last resort. It is not, after all, a magical solution that can transform you overnight. It is not a quick fix. Patients go through thorough evaluation, and preparation can take up to a year, or sometimes more.

One of the common misconceptions about undergoing weight loss surgery rather than losing the weight through diet and exercise is that you won't have to put in much effort. In reality, slowly increasing your activity level over time and slowly lowering your caloric intake over time will result in guaranteed fat loss.

But getting surgery does not mean you will automatically get the same benefits. By slowly increasing your daily activity, your muscles, tendons, and ligaments become stronger over time and will help you in your older age; something that will not happen through surgery.

Chapter 3:

Getting to Know Your Options

The idea of weight loss surgery is rooted in gastric surgery. This type of procedure is performed for patients who are suffering from severe ulcers and cancer. Gastric surgery involves the removal of a portion of the stomach and sometimes includes the small intestine. When we talk about bariatric surgery, there are basically two types of procedures involved, namely, malabsorptive surgeries and restrictive surgeries. Each provides a different approach to losing weight.

Restrictive Surgeries

This type of procedure involves reducing the size of the stomach so that the amount of food that can be eaten becomes restricted. For instance, a normal sized stomach can hold around three pints of solid food, but a restricted stomach may only be able to hold an ounce of food. However, a restricted stomach may eventually be able to hold two or three ounces of food, years after the surgery.

What doctors do, is create a small pouch by taking a small portion of the stomach. This pouch is placed at the end of the esophagus. Doctors leave a narrow opening from this pouch to the much larger part of the stomach. The pouch can hold around half an ounce, which is about the size of a shot glass. This small pouch has the ability to fill up quickly and empty slowly, which results in forcing the patient to eat less while giving the feeling of fullness.

Restrictive surgeries include gastric banding and vertical sleeve gastrectomy.

Gastric Banding

In this procedure, a band is placed around the top end of the patient's stomach. In the United States, there are two gastric banding devices that are commonly used and approved of by the FDA. These are, Realize band and LAP-BAND.

Gastric banding is considered to be minimally invasive. The surgeon only makes a small incision and neither the stomach, nor the intestine, has to be cut. This is why patients who choose gastric banding usually recover much faster, especially compared to those who undergo gastric bypass surgery.

Another advantage of gastric banding over other weight loss procedures is that it can be reversed easily. The surgeon will only need to remove the band surgically. Moreover, it is easier to control a patient's weight loss, as well as adjust to nutritional needs, with this procedure.

The band can be loosened or tightened and the process is simple enough that it can be done at the doctor's clinic. When there is a need to tighten, the band is injected with a saline solution. On the other hand, when it must be loosened, the doctor will remove the liquid using a needle.

It is also uncommon for gastric banding patients to experience serious complications. However, there is a possibility of the band slipping out of place, as well as possibly becoming too loose and allowing leakage. If any of these occur, corrective surgery may become necessary.

On the downside, the amount of weight lost via gastric banding may be less dramatic. On average, patients lose around 21 percent of their excess weight during the first year. In two years, patients usually lose an additional 26 percent of their excess weight. In ten years, the average weight loss is 13 percent.

Vertical Sleeve Gastrectomy

Another type of purely restrictive weight loss surgery is the vertical sleeve gastrectomy. This method is more invasive than gastric banding as it involves the removal of 75 percent of the stomach, using a vertical line of staples. This will turn the stomach into a sleeve, or a narrow tube, connected to the intestine.

Basically, it works to restrict the amount of food you can eat. Because the size of the stomach is significantly reduced, you can no longer eat as much as you want to, or used to, as the stomach can only hold so much.

This type of procedure is fairly new, as it was just introduced in 2011. However, because of its impressive results, it has emerged as one of the most sought after types of weight loss procedures.

Vertical sleeve gastrectomy works similar to gastric bypass. The big difference however, is that this procedure offers less disruption to the gastrointestinal tract. In this procedure, surgeons do not introduce a foreign element to the patient's body. This makes it a very enticing option, especially for individuals who are deemed unfit for gastric bypass surgery.

On the downside, vertical sleeve gastrectomy is a procedure that cannot be reversed. Its effects are permanent. Another downside is that some patients who are suffering from GERD, or heartburn, seem to slightly get worse after the surgery, though this does not happen to all patients. Moreover, this side effect seems to resolve itself in about 6 months to a year.

Malabsorptive Surgery

The second classification of weight loss surgery is called malabsorptive surgery. In this type of procedure, the small intestine is shortened. The connection of the stomach and the small intestine may also be altered.

As a result, the amount of food that is digested and absorbed in the stomach is significantly reduced, hence the term, malabsorptive. Both the process of digestion and absorption are passed on from the stomach to the small intestine.

There are two common types of malabsorptive surgery. These are gastric bypass and biliopancreatic diversion with duodenal switch.

Gastric Bypass

Just like in gastric banding, gastric bypass involves creating a small stomach pouch. Though while gastric banding allows food to pass through the pouch and on to the larger portion of the stomach for further digestion, gastric bypass makes the food enter the small pouch and directly passes it on to the small intestine.

How is this done?

For this to happen, the surgeon separates the small intestine from the larger portion of the stomach. One end of the small intestine is connected to the opening of the newly created small stomach pouch.

This procedure is one of the most sought after types of weight loss surgery, and with good reason. For one, it proves to offer the most dramatic weight loss. In fact, patients continue to lose weight 18 to 24 months after the procedure. There are patients whose weight loss is maintained at 60 to 70 percent, continuously, for as long as ten years.

Because of this, gastric bypass also proves helpful in treating weight related health conditions such as sleep apnea, high blood pressure, and diabetes. Ultimately, this kind of change offers patients an improved quality of life. It also shows to have a positive effect on their mental outlook.

But like other types of procedures, gastric bypass also has its share of disadvantages. Due to the fact that this procedure affects the way the digestive system processes and absorbs nutrients, there is a good chance of it leading to malnourishment. However, such can be prevented by taking the necessary supplements.

Patients who have undergone gastric bypass surgery are also at risk of developing gallstones due to their rapid weight loss. As mentioned earlier, dumping syndrome is another possible side effect, and is the reason why patients are advised against consuming foods that are rich in sugar.

The bottom line is, gastric bypass surgery can provide amazing results. But for that to happen, the patient also needs to commit to a permanent diet and lifestyle change. Otherwise, results will not be as promising and the surgery will be a waste of time and money.

Biliopancreatic Diversion with Duodenal Switch

This common weight loss procedure is complex and contains multiple parts. In this operation, a large portion of the stomach, as much as 80 percent, is removed. What remains of the stomach is the pyloric valve, which is responsible for releasing food into the small intestine. The small intestine is also cut and what remains is a limited portion that connects to the stomach.

As a result, the amount of food eaten and the amount of nutrients absorbed from food are both affected. Needless to say, it is certainly an effective weight loss procedure and is ideal for individuals with a BMI above 50, but it does come with risks.

Aside from possible complications from the surgery, a patient is likely to develop malnutrition and deficiencies. Patients are strongly advised to take supplements for the long term, in order to prevent such conditions.

Chapter 4:

Which Procedure for You?

After learning about the various options for a weight loss procedure, the question remains, how do you know which one is suitable for you? For this, you ultimately need to consult with your doctor in person. There is no amount of reading you can do that will substitute for an in-person evaluation. But for your own knowledge, here are a few pointers to help guide your decision-making process before you meet with a health professional:

Choose according to your weight loss goals.

Each type of weight loss procedure offers a different amount of weight loss per year and over the long-term. Gastric bypass patients, for instance, lose as much as 70 percent of their excess weight. So, if you are hoping for a more drastic change, this procedure is a promising option. Be mindful however, that rapid weight loss has its share of risks.

Gastric banding offers a less dramatic weight loss progression, at about 50 percent, while sleeve gastrectomy patients lose an average of 60 percent of their excess weight.

You should also keep in mind that the success of the procedure does not just depend on the work of the surgeon. You have to do your part as well. This means that you must comply to the diet and lifestyle changes that are recommended in order to achieve the best results, as well as to prevent the occurrence of serious complications from the surgery.

Do you want your weight loss to be drastic or gradual?

Your choice is also affected by your preferred rate of weight loss. If you want to achieve your expected weight loss goals within 12 to 15 months after the surgery, then opting for sleeve and gastric bypass may be a good idea. But if you want it slowly but surely, gastric banding may be a better option for you. This procedure offers a slower, yet steadier, weight loss rate and patients usually reach their weight loss goal in two years after the procedure.

Risks versus Proven Methods

Weight loss surgeries in general are relatively safe; their effectiveness has been proven. However, when it comes to supported research, gastric bypass and gastric banding are at an advantage over sleeve gastrectomy. This simply because sleeve gastrectomy is relatively new. Its safety and effectiveness is not as established as those procedures that have been around longer.

Do you have a fear of needles?

Gastric banding is not advised for patients with a fear of needles, as adjusting the band requires the use of needles. If you have this fear, it is something worth thinking about before you make your decision.

Permanent or Temporary?

Some people are more comfortable undergoing a reversible surgery because of the idea that what was placed in can be taken out. This is one reason that some people prefer gastric banding to other options. On the other hand, sleeve gastrectomy is a non-reversible procedure.

Less or More Invasive?

Gastric banding is the least invasive type of weight loss surgery; both gastric bypass and sleeve gastrectomy are more invasive. But according to experts, the percentage of complications is the same for all three operations.

Keep in mind that with the technology we have today, these procedures are relatively safe because of trial and error in the field.

How much are you willing to give up?

When you undergo weight loss surgery, you have to be willing to fully commit to what the operation requires. This can include the side effects as well as the diet and lifestyle changes that you must comply with.

Gastric banding requires continuous follow ups with the doctor for close monitoring in case there is a need to tighten or loosen the band. Both gastric banding and sleeve gastrectomy patients are less likely to experience dumping, while gastric bypass patients are likely to do so.

When eating foods that are high in sugar, gastric bypass patients will be immediately reminded that they have done something wrong. This reminder comes in the form of a racing heartbeat, dizziness, abdominal pain, profuse sweating, and/or diarrhea. On the upside, these possible effects can help to keep a patient's diet in check and contribute to the success of the weight loss process.

Sleeve gastrectomy and gastric banding patients will not feel the same side effects when they happen to have a taste of sugary foods. On the downside, they are on their own when it comes to following the recommended diet. They have to be disciplined enough to make the right food choices.

Finally, you need to seek the advice of your doctor and have yourself thoroughly evaluated so that your eligibility for your preferred procedure can be determined.

Three things that can help ensure the success of the operation.

First, you must be a viable candidate, which means you must comply with the criteria set for weight loss surgery patients. Second, you have to be fully committed. Third, you have to choose a competent surgeon.

So, how do you exactly choose a surgeon for your weight loss surgery?

There are 3 major criteria you can refer to, in order to ensure that you choose a competent surgeon.

One, you have to know how experienced the surgeon is in performing your preferred procedure. Needless to say, a more experienced surgeon has a better success rate than a less experienced one.

Two, the surgeon must be board certified. This is self-explanatory, however, it is not uncommon for people to go overseas and get their surgery done at an extremely discounted rate by a non-board certified surgeon. Ask yourself, is risking your future health worth saving a few thousand dollars?

Three, you must determine the level of support the surgeon and the entire staff is willing to provide after the surgery. After all, you do not just need the surgeon during the operation. You need guidance, before, during and especially after the surgery.

Make sure your surgeon can provide the kind of professional support that you require and don't be afraid to ask for as much help as you need, as you are the one paying for the service, and they are there to help you. Confidence and trust in the surgeon and the entire staff can be established by asking questions. Get to know the surgeon by asking the right questions. Testimonials from other patients are especially helpful and can erase any doubt that you might have had.

What else should you expect from surgery?

One of the most important things you must pay attention to after your surgery is the way you eat. For the first two days after the surgery, you will be placed on a liquid-only diet. This means that you are only allowed to consume milk, broth, unsweetened juice, sugar-free gelatin and strained cream soup.

The second phase of your diet, which usually lasts for two to four weeks, involves pureed foods. You can puree solid food such as fish, lean ground meats, egg whites, fruits, and vegetables, by blending them with water, broth, sugar-free juice, etc. At this stage, it may be safe to steer clear from dairy products and spices, depending on your doctor's recommendation.

Based on your doctor's advice, you may be able to switch to the third phase, which involves soft, solid foods. Examples include cooked vegetables, soft and fresh fruits, as well as ground or diced meats. After eight weeks, it may be alright to start switching to solid foods.

Even many weeks after the surgery, you should avoid eating breads, tough meats, granola, dried fruits, popcorn, fibrous fruits and vegetables, carbonated drinks, nuts, and seeds; otherwise, you are likely to suffer from gastrointestinal symptoms.

This overview of your nutrition post-surgery is a mere outline for what you can expect. At the end of the day, you must seek the guidance of your doctor and follow his/her protocol. This way, you will avoid developing serious complications and only get the best results from your operation!

Conclusion

I worked hard on creating the best guide for bariatric surgery that I could. Hopefully it helped you with deciding on whether or not you'd like to pursue the idea of surgery to aid in your weight loss journey. Maybe it also motivated you to start shedding those extra pounds without the help of surgery. Regardless, if you are interested, check with your doctor and dietician before you get started and don't be afraid to share this book with someone who might be able to use it.

If you feel like you learned something from this book, please take the time to share your thoughts with me by sending me a message. I would also appreciate it if you left a review on Amazon!

Thank you and good luck in your journey!

18288187R00038

Printed in Great Britain
by Amazon